stuttering and your child:
questions and answers

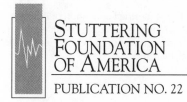

STUTTERING
FOUNDATION
OF AMERICA

PUBLICATION NO. 22

stuttering and your child: questions and answers

First Printing—1989
Second Printing—1990
Third Printing—1991
Fourth Printing—1994
Fifth Printing—1996

Published by

Stuttering Foundation of America
P.O. Box 11749
Memphis, Tennessee 38111-0749

Library of Congress Catalog No. 90-195655
ISBN 0-933388-28-4

To Parents, Teachers, and All Those Concerned With Stuttering in the Young Child

This book represents the most up-to-date thoughts of seven leading authorities in the field of stuttering. All attach great importance to early intervention in the prevention of stuttering in the young child. Their names are listed below.

You will find answers to the questions most often asked by parents who are concerned about stuttering and their child. These answers will enable you, the reader, to work with the child in a positive way and thus to contribute significantly to the healthy and normal development of fluency.

Jane Fraser
President

Stuttering Foundation of America

Edward G. Conture, Ph.D., Syracuse University
Richard F. Curlee, Ph.D., University of Arizona
Hugo H. Gregory, Ph.D., Northwestern University
Barry Guitar, Ph.D., University of Vermont
Lois A. Nelson, Ph.D., University of Wisconsin
William H. Perkins, Ph.D., University of Southern California
Dean E. Williams, Ph.D., University of Iowa

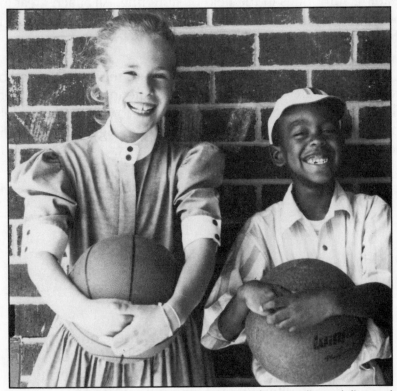

photo credit: paul diamond

Contents

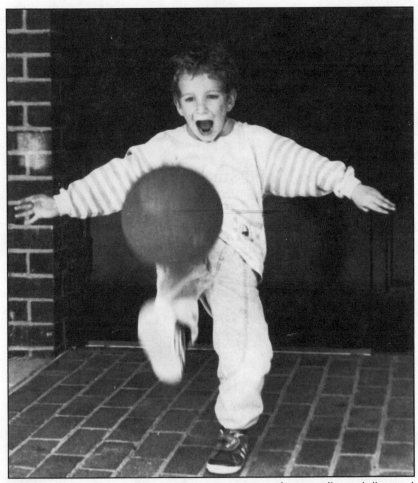

photo credit: paul diamond

Chapter 1

does my child stutter?

Richard F. Curlee, Ph.D.
Professor, Dept. Speech and Hearing Sciences
University of Arizona

He may. Many children do begin to stutter during their pre-school years. This chapter answers some of the questions that parents often ask when they become concerned about their child's speech. As you read on and find out more about stuttering, you should be better able to answer this question.

What is "normal" speech?

"Normal" is what most of us hope that we and our children are, and what many of us think that we are seeing and hearing on TV. In fact, "normal" speech reflects a wide range of abilities. Some people speak barely above a whisper, others at a high volume. Some talk so rapidly that if you talk to them you can hardly get a word in edgewise. Still others hesitate and revise, repeat words and phrases "um" and "ah", and seem as if they are never going to finish their point. Most of us fall somewhere in between.

So, how can you tell if your child has crossed the line between "normal" and "abnormal"? First, it is important to remember that there isn't a line. Second, what's "normal" always represents someone's judgment. If you are concerned about your child's speech, that means that you must have made a judgment that he or she may not be "normal". It may be that your standards of "normal" are too closely pegged to the superior speech that you observe from professional TV performers. As you read on and find out more about stuttering, you will be able to decide if your expectations for your child's speech have been unrealistic or if you need to seek an evaluation of your child's speech from an expert in your area.

What is stuttering?

Stuttering is an involuntary repetition, prolongation or blockage of a word or part of a word that a person is trying to say. Children who stutter know what they want to say. They may have said it hundreds, even thousands, of times before without stuttering. Yet, this time, in spite of all of their efforts, they are unable to say the word smoothly, effortlessly.

When children who stutter attempt to push through these involuntary disruptions of their speech, they often begin to avert their eyes, bob their heads and, in other ways, struggle with speaking. Struggling to speak often does not begin until after a child has been stuttering for awhile. Even though a child's use of force to speak fluently is well-intentioned, it does much more harm than good and generally indicates that professional help is needed.

How can you recognize it?

In its initial stages, stuttering can be difficult to recognize because most children beginning to stutter often sound a lot like other children their age much of the time. At first, a child may only stutter occasionally. Stuttering occurs in some situations but not in others, often with no apparent rhyme or reason. Several days, perhaps a week or so, may go by with no problems. Then, without warning, a child may go through a period when he seems to stutter every time he opens his mouth.

There are several things you can look for in trying to determine if your child is beginning to stutter or is just fumbling around talking like many other children his age. Children who stutter seem to have special problems getting words started, and many of these disruptions occur at the beginning of sentences. When they stutter, they also tend to repeat parts of words, e.g., sounds or syllables, rather than whole words or phrases. In addition, they frequently repeat the portions of words two or more times before they are able to say what they want. Sometimes a child may give exaggerated, prolonged stress to a sound in a word, or seem to be stuck with no sound or word coming out, or seem to be working hard at speaking, or look away just as his speech is disrupted. All of these are signs of stuttering, and if you observe your child talking this way, you should make an appointment for him to see someone in your area who specializes in helping those who stutter.

When does stuttering typically begin?

A child's risk for beginning to stutter increases from about his 2nd until his 4th birthday, then decreases gradually until about the age twelve. Often, stuttering begins gradually during the period when a child is acquiring language at a rapid rate. It rarely begins until after a child is speaking in short meaningful phrases. In fact, most kids who stutter have been using sentences for some time, giving their parents no reason to suspect that they may not be developing speech normally before they begin to stutter.

Most people who are ever going to stutter will have begun before they reach their 5th birthday. Practically no one begins after age twelve unless they suffer a serious head injury. So, stuttering is really a developmental problem of childhood.

Is stuttering a common problem?

There are more than 45 million people in the world today who stutter, and approximately three million live in the United States. It is more common than cleft palate but less common than delayed speech development. Indeed, it occurs often enough that most of us have had some experience with a neighbor, classmate, co-worker, or family member who stutters.

About 5% of all children are likely to stutter for several months or more at some time during their lives. Because stuttering runs in families, it is much more common in some families than others. For example, if a father or mother has ever stuttered, the chances that their children will stutter are three to five times greater than that for families in which neither parent has ever stuttered.

Stuttering is most prevalent among preschoolers, but decreases among older age groups. Nationwide, across all age groups, about seven persons in every thousand stutter. Among adults, about three in a thousand stutter severely and feel that their educational, vocational and social achievements have been affected by stuttering. In contrast, there are many prominent, successful people who have stuttered throughout most of their lives. Winston Churchill stuttered; so did Sir Isaac Newton, King George VI of England and writers Somerset Maughman and Budd Schulberg. So, too, do Bruce Willis, Carly Simon, Bob Love, and James Earle Jones.

Does stuttering look and sound the same in all children?

No more than any other two people look and sound alike. One dramatic way in which young stutterers may differ is the way in which their speaking difficulties begin. As was noted earlier, stuttering typically begins gradually with periods of occasional stuttering interspersed with periods of completely normal-sounding speech. For a few children, stuttering begins with obvious physical tensions and struggle, jaw tremors, frustration, even tears.

If stuttering persists, the nature of the child's speech disruptions often change. Some may begin to exhibit eye blinks, lip tremors, or head jerks during their speech disruptions. Often, such behavior disappears with time, gradually, just as it originally appeared. Other children may react to their speech disruptions with a great deal of frustration. These children are apt to avoid talking or even participating in situations where they think they might stutter. In time, their efforts to avoid stuttering are likely to become more of a problem than their disfluent speech ever

Things parents can do to help the child who stutters.

1) Listen patiently to what your child says, not how it is said. Respond to the message rather than the stuttering.
2) Allow your child to complete her thoughts without interrupting.
3) Keep natural eye contact while your child is talking.
4) Avoid filling in or speaking your child's thoughts or ideas. Let the words be her own.
5) After your child speaks, reply slowly and unhurriedly, using some of the same words.
   For example, if she says, "I s-s-see the b-b-b-bunny." You reply in an easy relaxed way, "oh yes, you see the bunny. He's cute."
6) Wait a second or so before responding to your child. This helps to calm and slow things down and should help her speech.
7) Spend at least 5 minutes each day devoted to talking with your child in an unhurried, easy, relaxed manner.
8) Find ways to show your child that you love and value her and that you enjoy your time together.

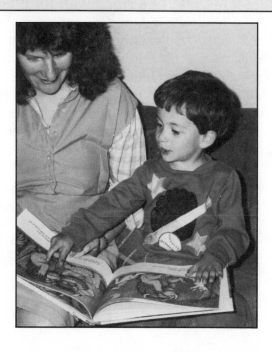

could be. Without help, their anticipation and fear of stuttering can create a barrier which prevents them from doing what they are capable of doing.

Why does he stutter some times and not others?

Among young children especially, stuttering is very inconsistent. The amount and type of stuttering can vary from one day to another, from one situation to another. It can even vary during the same conversation. No one knows why stuttering is so inconsistent. We do know that stuttering often increases significantly when children are excited, excessively tired, apprehensive, feel rushed to talk or on display. Most of us, in fact, probably become more disfluent at such times. Occasionally, however, a young child will stutter severely, for no apparent reason, under the most calm, tranquil circumstances. One of the reasons that stuttering has continued to puzzle experts over the years is such seemingly unpredictable changes in its frequency and severity.

Is stuttering something he's stuck with for life?

Probably not. Most children who begin to stutter gradually stop–perhaps as many as 80%. In fact, nearly half stop within a year of beginning to stutter. Of those children who continue to stutter as adults, about a third may stutter severely enough to adversely affect educational or vocational achievements. But even adults with chronic, severe stuttering problems can be helped to speak so that routine everyday communication is not a significant problem.

If your child has just begun to stutter, the odds are strongly in favor of his stopping. If he has been stuttering for some time, if he appears to struggle with his speech disfluencies, avoids talking in some situations or has expressed concern about his speech, you probably should seek professional assistance. Persistent, consistent stuttering is unlikely to disappear with age unless he receives therapy for his problem.

Chapter 2

why does my child stutter?

Edward G. Conture, Ph.D.
Professor, Department of Communication
Sciences and Disorders
Syracuse University

The question most frequently asked by parents is "Why does my child stutter"? No one knows for sure but it makes perfect sense that parents want to know. It would seem that if "the cause" of stuttering could be identified, steps could be taken to eliminate it. The fact is that we do not need to answer that question in order to help your child.

What determines whether a child stutters?

While stuttering is often thought to have one cause it may actually have several. Stuttering probably begins when a combination of factors come together. For different young stutterers, different things may lead to the same end: stuttering. Searching for one "cause" when several exist may become part of the problem rather than its solution.

There are many theories why children stutter, but none satisfactorily account for all that is known about stuttering. Children who stutter are no more apt to have psychological problems than children who don't stutter. Children who stutter are no more anxious than average. There is also no reason to believe that stuttering usually results from some emotional trauma or abnormal child rearing practice.

There is reason to believe, however, that for some children a predisposition to stutter may be transmitted genetically, even though it is also apparent that certain environmental conditions have to be present for stuttering to develop in some if not all children. The speech mechanism of these children appears to be vulnerable to disruptions in the flow of speech. The cause of such vulnerability is presently unknown but some scientists now believe that some slight brain dysfunction disrupts the precise coordination of the 100 or more muscles used to produce speech. Furthermore, there is also reason to believe that some children may react to such speech disruptions with apprehension and tension, making them worse, and increasing the likelihood that their stuttering will persist.

What causes stuttering? What keeps it going?

Things that **cause** stuttering may be, and probably are, quite different from things that **keep it going, aggravate** or **worsen** it. For example, if you mishandle a knife, you may cut your finger. The knife **causes** the cut and initial pain. Salt rubbed into the cut makes the pain continue or even worsen but the salt does not cause the cut.

We still haven't found the "knife" that causes stuttering. However, we do know something about the "salt" that keeps it going, makes it worse or aggravates it. Indeed, we will focus more on those things that keep stuttering going than on the things that may have started or initially caused it because you can do something about these things, you can **change** these things that keep stuttering going.

Who is to blame?

Parents are not to blame for stuttering. After years of study, we have found no reason to believe that the way parents rear their child has a significant influence on stuttering.

On the other hand there are things that parents and the rest of the family can **do** that **help** the child's speech; for example, they can try to provide a calmer, less hurried lifestyle in the home; they can speak less hurriedly when talking to their child; they can allow their child to finish his thoughts; they can pause a second or so before responding to their child's questions; they can try not to talk for their child, and so forth.

Unfortunately, there are also things that parents, brothers, sisters, aunts and uncles and the rest of the family **do** that **hinder** the child's speech, for example, finishing the child's sentences, interrupting the child while he is talking, encouraging or requiring him to talk rapidly, speaking to the child using a rapid rate of speech, maintaining an overly rapid lifestyle within the home.

None of the things a listener or parent do that may hinder a child's fluent speech make that individual a bad person or parent. However, these types of behavior make it **difficult** for a child who is already having trouble establishing his speech fluency. If parents change some things in the home (for example, slowing down their rate of speech, decreasing the number of times they ask the child to perform for or give little plays or speeches to people visiting the home), they can do a lot to help.

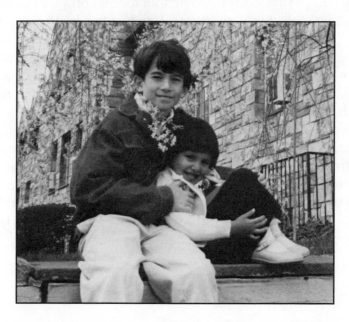

What part do the child's abilities play?

A big part. The huge Clydesdale horses that pull the Bud-weiser beer wagon have little hope of winning the Kentucky Derby, no matter how much encouragement they receive from their owners! Simply put, from birth, both horses and people have certain skills and abilities that are unique to them and on which environmental factors have little or no influence.

Each child has his or her strengths and weaknesses; even within one family, each child may be very different. And, after all, wouldn't it be a boring world, if we were all the same? Parents need to realize that each of their children has unique abilities and that some of these may be influenced very little by things you as parents may do (even though, as we said above, there are some things that you do that can help or hinder the child's development of fluent speech).

Do problems with the brain cause stuttering?

Since the brain is involved with speaking, researchers have long been trying to find out whether the anatomy (structure) and function (activity) of stutterers' brains differ from people who don't stutter. Modern advances in technology, for example, brain imaging procedures, now permit clearer, more precise viewing of brain activity and structure. A recent oral report of a brain imaging study indicates that there may be subtle differences in the brain activity and/or structure of *some* adult stutterers. How-ever, there is no published evidence to show how, or if, these differences influence stutterers' actual speaking behavior; fur-thermore, there is no published evidence to show that these differences *cause* stuttering. We hope that with continued ad-vances in technology, we should know more about the role the brain plays in stuttering but we don't have to wait for this knowl-edge in order to help your child.

Things That HELP

(1) Provide a calmer, less-hurried life style in the home.
(2) Speak less hurriedly when talking to the child.
(3) Allow the child to finish his thoughts.
(4) Try not to talk for the child or rush him to finish his thoughts.
(5) Pause a second or so before responding to the child's questions or comments.
(6) Turn off the television and radio during dinner time; this is a time for family conversation not listening to television or radio programs.
(7) If your child begins to talk to you while you are doing things that require concentration (for example, driving a car, using a knife to cut vegetables) tell him that you can't look away right now but that you are listening to him and that he has your attention.

Things that HINDER

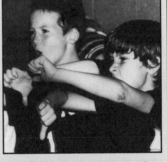

(1) Finishing the child's sentences.
(2) Rushing the child to finish his thoughts or sentences.
(3) Interrupting the child while he is talking.
(4) Encouraging or requiring him to talk rapidly, precisely and maturely at all times.
(5) Frequently correcting, criticizing, or trying to change the way he talks, or pronounces sounds or words.
(6) Speaking to the child using a rapid rate of speech, especially when telling him to slow his own rate of speaking down.
(7) Maintaining an overly rapid lifestyle within the home (or constantly feeling or acting as if "every thing had to be done yesterday").
(8) Making him give little speeches, plays or read aloud to visiting friends, relatives or neighbors.

Can a child "catch" stuttering?

Hardly. Stuttering is not a problem that is spread like a disease or common cold. Stuttering "germs" aren't floating around in the air, swimming in the water supply or resting on doorknobs just waiting for us to breath or drink them in or pick them up on our hands. No, developing a stuttering problem is far more complex.

If my child "imitates" someone else's stuttering, will he become a stutterer?

We've never heard of one crow, mynah bird, mockingbird or parrot–all famous imitators–who began to stutter through living with and imitating a stutterer! Further, as mentioned above, normally fluent speech clinicians who have worked with literally hundreds of individuals who stutter haven't–through all their exposure to stuttering–either "picked-up" or developed the problem. Most stutterers began stuttering without ever having heard anyone else stutter.

The imitation myth dies hard, however, so too did the one about warts on your hands from handling frogs and toads. In part, its refusal to die relates to our belief that children copy the habits of their elders like so many little copy machines. While this copying may be at least partially true for certain behaviors, it's hard to figure how this works with stuttering when none of the people the child communicates with are stutterers, a situation more common than not.

Why do some children begin to stutter after a fairly normal period of speech and language development?

Some children who stutter struggle with their speech and language right from the beginning while others seemingly have little trouble with speech until they start to stutter. Most, however, only start stuttering after they have begun to use sentences to express their ideas (sometime after 2 years of age). No one knows for sure why some children begin to stutter after a period of seemingly normal speech development. One idea is that the various abilities a child needs for speaking develop at different rates. For example, it is not uncommon to find a child whose expressive language skills are quite superior but whose ability to speak with clarity, speed and precision is quite delayed. Perhaps this sort of developmental "mismatch" contributes to difficulties some children have maintaining smooth, easy speech after they have been talking normally for awhile. Whatever the case, while stuttering is often described as a "disorder of childhood," it is a disorder that typically emerges sometime after the beginning of childhood speech development.

Do children stutter on purpose?

In our experience this only happens when one child is ridiculing or mocking another child by overtly imitating the other child's stutterings. It is not fun to stutter and few children appear interested or willing to do so if they have any choice in the matter.

It is possible, however, to think of two exceptions to the rule: (1) a child seeking parental attention (this is based on the premise that any attention is better than no attention at all) and (2) a child verbally "acting out" against the parents for some reason. But these possibilities are quite rare. Simply put, we know of no documented evidence to support claims that youngsters stutter on purpose. Instead, our clinical experience working with many, many of these children and their families is that if children who stutter could or would do anything on purpose, it would be to speak more fluently.

Does stuttering begin after a sudden trauma?

For most children who stutter, the onset of stuttering, as well as its recovery, appears to be gradual. Stuttering rarely begins after a sudden trauma.

Occasionally, however, a child will have a very serious fright or injury or unexpected experience just before stuttering begins.

However, and this must be stressed, these types of sudden traumatic onsets of stuttering are very few and far between. In fact, most children who experience these sorts of sudden traumas or shocks DO NOT begin to stutter.

Can stuttering be caused by moving?

It's been said that you can go 3000 miles and still remain where you are. Indeed the heaviest baggage you take with you when you travel is yourself. You may be moving to new surroundings but your old self and problems still follow you. The same goes for your child.

First, every year many families move across town, across or out of state without having their children begin or develop stuttering. Second, if moving were such a powerful influence on stuttering, we'd see much more stuttering, which we don't, in the children of families of people that work in the army. Third, we must once again distinguish between what causes and what worsens it. For example, let's assume the child's speech was already slow in its development and the child, for whatever reason, began to get concerned about meeting and making new friends, leaving old ones, and the like. If this were the case, the stage might be set for conditions that would disrupt fluent speech. The chances for disruptions increase even more if the child is tired because of the packing, the trip to the new house, and unpacking. Further, if the parents themselves–who are just as tired as their children or even more so–react to the move by becoming fatigued, overly stressed and unpleasant to be around, then the child may find it hard or unpleasant to talk with them. In this way, the move may aggravate an already existing or emerging problem. But by itself, moving does not cause stuttering.

Why do more boys stutter than girls?

About three times as many boys as girls stutter; however, boys are more apt than girls to have other speech and language problems too. This apparent difference in susceptibility to stuttering has been attributed to differences in boys' and girls' biological constitution, physical maturation, and/or speech and language development, as well as to gender differences in parents' attitudes and expectations. The evidence is not sufficient for us to rule out any of these possible explanations with confidence.

Can starting school cause stuttering?

Beginning school is a time of excitement, a time of new challenges for all children. The young child must meet and deal with new friends and adults and learn to work and play in new surroundings. It is a time of uncertainty for all children as new relationships are being made, new skills tried out, and new rules being learned. While these events may make it hard for the young child to keep all his previous advances in speech development, they don't cause stuttering.

Once again, the excitement, the uncertainty and the stresses to perform that occur during the new school year may aggravate an existing or developing problem like salt rubbed into a wound. However, your child's future lies with his friends as much as with his elders and school is an excellent place for him to learn how to deal with people his own age. You can be of tremendous help to your child by supporting him as he learns how to play and work with other children at school.

Can too much excitement cause stuttering?

It's been said that too much of a good thing is no good. Excitement, which we all feel at various times, can be wonderfully stimulating but for a young child, too much excitement for too long can be too much. While excited, the child may continuously run around inside and outside the house until dropping with fatigue, all the while jabbering away a 100 miles an hour. Very few parents could remain fluent if they acted like this!

No, excitement doesn't cause stuttering but it can make it difficult for the young child to continue to speak fluently, particularly when he is talking fast while tired and competing with other talkers. We don't want our children to vegetate in the corner like a mushroom nor do we want them to continually speed around like a bullet. Parents can and should help their child bring the excitement level down by quietly playing with him while speaking slowly themselves with a quiet tone of voice. If you try to be reasonably relaxed and not do things or speak in a hurry, it really helps your child to do the same.

Does my child stutter because of nervousness?

There is no evidence to prove that children who stutter are more nervous more often than usual nor is there evidence to suggest that nervousness is the reason why children stutter, though it may aggravate the problem. Your child doesn't stutter because he is a nervous person but when required to speak maturely, precisely and quickly, he may feel under stress. Children can't be reared in cocoons or like delicate house plants; they have to be allowed to get excited, nervous or tired as the situation dictates. These children, like all children, will experience situations in which they'll get more nervous than usual. You can look for ways to help your child deal with these situations constructively and successfully.

A parting shot

This section examined various theories that nerves, excitement, trauma, beginning school, imitation and the like cause stuttering. What these various theories all seem to share in common is a tendency to provide a simple solution to a complex problem. Most of these theories also seem to blur the distinction between things that make stuttering worse and those things which may actually cause it in the first place. This section should help you understand the distinction between the two; other sections will discuss in more detail things that you can change to help your child. If you can focus on what you can do in the present and future rather than concentrating on what may have happened in the past, you can be of tremendous help to your child.

Chapter 3

how does our home life influence his stuttering?

Lois A. Nelson, Ph.D.
Professor, Department of Communicative Disorders
University of Wisconsin - Madison

Should we treat him like our other children?

Yes, of course–with some exceptions. Your child should think of himself as a "regular kid," a regular kid who just happens to stutter. To do this, he needs to be taught the standards of behavior, the social values, and the kinds of responsibility that you expect of your other children. Children are not helped to feel "regular" if they receive special treatment whether the special treatment is because they stutter or for any other reason. On the other hand, you probably know that your own children differ from each other in many ways. Many parents comment that they discipline each child a little differently. They may problem-solve with one child but insist on a strict follow-the-rules system with another. They have discovered through experience that strategies which work with one child may be less effective with another.

What are some exceptions?

We know that the child who stutters may take more time to talk, and we hope you will try to be patient and listen until he finishes. You should try to ensure that the child has opportunities to express his ideas. Nevertheless, a child who stutters can learn to take turns talking and develop other social skills as well. Stuttering should not become an excuse for him to monopolize the conversation or interrupt the person who is talking.

Do we expect too much from our child?

Sometimes parents expect too much from their child. Children can feel pressured if they try, yet frequently fail, to meet the family's expectations. Likewise, a child feels pressured if he does not live up to his own expectations. This kind of stress can aggravate stuttering.

Should we leave him with a babysitter?

Some children have a more difficult time than others when separated from their parents for an afternoon or evening. As much as possible, this decision should be made separately from the fact that your child stutters. Would you leave him with a sitter if he didn't stutter? If the answer is "yes," then feel free to leave him with the sitter.

You will probably instruct the sitter about house rules, bedtime routines, and leave a telephone number where you can be reached. Similarly, you can prepare the sitter on how to handle the situation if your child stutters. Calmly inform her ahead of time that your child may stutter and briefly describe how his stuttering sounds. Use descriptive terms such as "he repeats the first syllable of a word" or "he has trouble getting the word started". Explain whatever it is the child actually does most of the time. Since children often feel uncomfortable when they know they are being discussed, try to do this when the child is not present. If he happens to overhear you talking about his stuttering, he may feel that something is amiss. At that point, it would be wise to talk with him about it openly.

Then tell her what you say and do when your child stutters; for example, "we wait for him to say the word himself and try not to finish words or sentences for him; we try not to cut him off or get him to talk less; we don't imitate his stuttering or tease him; and we look at him as he talks". You could explain the situations in which he is likely to stutter more, such as when he gets really excited, overly tired, is hurried or is asked many questions. Ask the sitter to be patient and listen to what he says, not how he says it and respond to that.

What Babysitters Can Do to Help.

1) Treat the child who stutters like all the other children you babysit.
2) Don't let him get away with things that his brothers and sisters aren't allowed to do.
3) Here are a few "don'ts" that will help:
    a) don't hurry the child's speech
    b) don't finish words or sentences for him
    c) don't interrupt
    d) don't correct pronunciations
    e) don't keep the child from talking
4) Be patient and pay attention to what the child says, not how he says it. Respond to the message.

Does he need more rest than other children?

He may. Most of us make more mistakes in pronouncing words and expressing ideas clearly when we are tired, distressed or distracted. If fatigue appears to influence your child's speech, you may want to make doubly sure that he gets sufficient rest.

Does your family's life style need to be changed?

Many parents find that their young child's stuttering increases when the family's life style is fast-paced. Children differ considerably in their energy levels and the effect that a hurried family life style has on them. Be guided by the unique nature of your child and if slowing down the family's pace seems to help your child, then it is important for you to do.

Should my child have regular bedtime hours?

Consistency in bedtime helps any child adjust to a sleep schedule. Consistency also has value from another perspective. Children benefit from the order of daily routine: waking, dressing, mealtimes, and going to bed. They learn what to expect in their lives and when to expect it. This kind of structure reduces uncertainty in their lives. Of course, parents shouldn't be expected to follow an overly rigid schedule. Use your best judgment in making these decisions.

Does my child who stutters need more attention?

Whether your child continually seeks, wants or needs additional attention depends partly on his feelings of self-worth, his personality, and his ability to entertain himself. Children value individual time with a parent. If your child stutters often, extra attention and listening time are likely to help him feel better about the talking he does and about his importance to you. Opportunity for uninterrupted listening time can markedly decrease stuttering in very young children. When a child expects to be and is interrupted by brothers and sisters, it's difficult for him to talk fluently. He feels pressured to talk quickly when he has to continually compete for Mom's and Dad's attention.

Do I let him watch overly-exciting TV shows?

We hope not, particularly if he is a preschooler. Many young children are easily excited by what they see and hear and some shows actually frighten them. High excitement levels, from any source, may increase stuttering in children. Long after a child's speech has improved, he is still likely to stutter occasionally when he is under stress or highly excited. Parents tell us, "He is really talking well now. The only time he still stutters is when he gets excited." If a television show or any other experience is too exciting for him, then it is too exciting for any of your other children as well.

Should we watch what he eats?

Children need a balanced diet in order to grow and be healthy. Your child's physician, public health nurses and hospital dieticians are excellent sources of information about adequate nutrition. Follow their advice and your own good judgment.

What if my child is frequently inattentive and hyperactive?

Some children exhibit behavior that parents and teachers describe as chronically restless, impulsive, or distractible–to name only a few traits. These parents express concern that their child is truly inattentive as well as hyperactive. They also express the fear that this may hinder him both academically and socially. They find that their child's behavior frequently disrupts their home life and report that their efforts to cope with him are only partially effective. A few children who exhibit the above traits also stutter and the parents worry that the hyperactivity contributes to the stuttering and vice versa. If you are concerned about your child's inattentiveness and/or hyperactivity, you should contact your family physician or pediatrician and request that your child be evaluated by specialists in the area of Attention Deficit Disorder (ADD). If this diagnosis is made, then medical management precedes or at least should take place simultaneously with speech therapy. Many states have a support group for parents or children with attention deficit problems.

How neat should his room be?

It's not neatness in itself that is important here. It's how your child feels about keeping his room neat. How does your child respond to the reminders to pick up his things? Does he feel that you are nagging him? Does he feel pressured to comply? Most parents comment that they wonder if he's ever going to learn to be neat. Most children react to those reminders or comments with no observable effect on their speech or other behavior. Listen to what he says and how fluently he says it. Does he stutter more frequently or more severely whenever the appearance of his room is discussed? You may be more willing to re-evaluate your priorities about neatness if you discover that continually nagging him about neatness contributes to stuttering.

What about fighting with other children?

Fighting seems to be part of learning to live with brothers and sisters and the neighborhood kids. Much as parents dislike it, children do and say mean things to each other. It's a reality. Children who stutter are just as likely to do and say mean things as other children. Some fighting among children is to be expected and parents should not be overly concerned about this.

What about fights and arguments between his mother and father?

Arguments between parents occur even in families where the father and mother have a very good relationship. Professionals such as psychologists and family counselors consider it important for children to discover that disagreements do not signal a loss of love or an impending divorce. They want the children to learn that arguing with someone doesn't diminish that person's caring for them.

But when verbal fighting between adults is chronic or becomes excessive or abusive, children can become alarmed. They feel vulnerable in these situations, and they are. Older children may be forced into the role of protector for one parent or peacemaker for the family. This kind of environment does not nurture the child's development. If fights and arguments in your family affect your child's stuttering, and you have been unsuccessful in coping with the problem, seek help from professionals, such as family counseling agencies.

His mother and father are thinking about separating. Will this aggravate his stuttering?

Perhaps, but it all depends on how the parents and child react. It may also affect many other things, such as his performance at school, playing with friends and so forth. But if the relationship between his parents is already generating friction within the family, it may already have aggravated his stuttering. What seems to be important is how the child reacts to the current family problem and what he expects to happen to him if his parents do separate. Do what you can to maintain stability in his life as well as your own.

His mother and father are separated or divorced. Will this hurt his stuttering?

Separation and divorce in American families is not unusual. Although you may be especially concerned about your child who stutters, the emotional impact of the events leading to that decision will have influenced the entire family. Reassure your children that they are loved, that they didn't cause the break and that both parents will always remain their parents. Keep in mind that usually no single event in a child's life is responsible for maintaining stuttering.

I am a single parent. Does this influence his stuttering?

One main difference is that a single parent simply has no one with whom to share the stresses of daily living. Many single parents do a good job of coping with these demands and this has a very good impact on the child. The ways in which a parent deals effectively with stress are likely to be ones the child learns to use in handling his own.

Should anyone in the family correct his stuttering?

No. That doesn't really help. Even if the family member has the best intentions, the child who stutters seldom reacts to correcting as kind and helpful. He may get the message that he is not acceptable unless he speaks well. After all, if he were okay, why would everyone be trying to change the way he talks?

Should we let his younger or older brother and sister imitate his stuttering?

No. Imitation is a form of teasing. It hurts anyone when they are teased, especially when it's about behavior they cannot help doing. When teasing occurs, you can tell your children that imitating their brother's stuttering actually makes it harder for him to talk and might even make his stuttering worse. But do not scold them for teasing and try to realize that you cannot stop teasing entirely and that you should not get overly concerned about it.

Should we have the TV, radio or stereo on during meal times?

Definitely not. Children generally find it more difficult to talk when there is a lot of activity going on or when the radio, TV or stereo is being played in the same room. Background noise, music or speech forces the child into a form of competition and can contribute to breakdowns in his speech.

Meal times can be quite hectic with brothers and sisters verbally competing for Mom's and Dad's attention. Children are bursting with things to tell and wanting to be heard. Parents find their attention divided between listening to their children and eating their food! If parents' attention is further divided by TV or radio programs, a child will quickly sense that his parents' interest is focussed elsewhere and that they are only half-heartedly listening to him. Children react to such inattention, and it can contribute to their stuttering. Turn off the radio, TV and stereo during meals. This will improve the situation and talking during meal times will be less stressful and competitive for everyone, particularly the child who may stutter. Mealtimes should be one of the best times for sharing the day's experiences and having an enjoyable exchange of ideas.

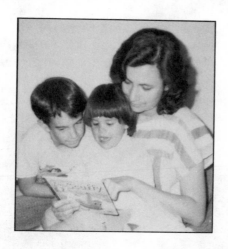

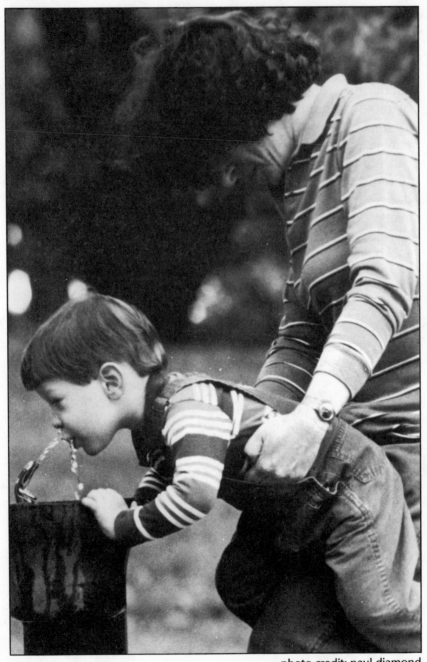

photo credit: paul diamond

Chapter 4

what do I tell people about my child's stuttering?

Dean E. Williams, Ph.D.
Professor Emeritus,
Department of Speech Pathology and Audiology
University of Iowa

It helps when discussing stuttering with a child to explain it by using analogies taken from common experiences in his every day life. This approach enables the child to view stuttering not as something mysterious and scary but as something understandable and solvable. It also provides a common platform from which you and your child can understand what each is talking about. Such mutual understanding helps to get the child on a positive course for coping with his speech problem. Your child is learning new things every day. We know, but sometimes forget, that making mistakes is an essential part of learning. He can be helped to understand that he made mistakes when he learned to dress himself, when he learned to eat with a spoon, when he learned his A B Cs, or to count, etc., etc. But, the mistakes were okay. They were a normal part of learning.

Learning to talk is a big job for a little person. It's very important with young children to view the stuttering as "making mistakes." He is repeating sound and words. That's alright. Everyone makes mistakes as they learn to talk. Some make more than others–just as some children make more mistakes than others as they learn to count, or, to read, or to catch a ball, and so forth.

(Examples used should correspond to your child's own interests.) Your child is probably making more mistakes than many children when he talks, but probably not as many as some of his friends as he learns other things. It helps to have this pointed out to him. His speech will undoubtedly develop all right. In the meantime, its helpful to reassure your child that it's okay to make mistakes–that it is much more important to you that he talks and has fun talking. If he does this, it then will be easy for you to learn the things he thinks about, the way he feels, and the things he likes and doesn't like. You can assure him that these are the important things about talking–not whether he makes mistakes as he learns how to talk.

If your child is not only repeating sound but also is tensing and struggling, you can follow the same kind of explanation as outlined above. However, there will be a need to add to the examples.

Let us say as an illustration that a child is learning to catch a ball. He's dropping the ball quite a bit. He doesn't like doing this, so he begins to tense up and "pounce" at the ball. He begins to drop it more often. He is now trying hard "not to drop it." The same thing occurs when one begins to learn to ride a bicycle. Often the child will tense up to try "not to fall off." He will fall off more often. In a sense these children are "fighting the making of mistakes." The same thing can happen if a child begins to believe he should not make mistakes while talking. In an effort to "not" make them, he physically tenses and struggles. This only makes talking more difficult. He can be helped to see that it is more beneficial to "go ahead and talk and stutter easily." This makes it easier for him to say what he wants to say.

What do I tell his brothers and his sisters about stuttering and about what they can do to help?

You can explain stuttering to his brothers and sisters in much the same way as you explain it to your child. He can be present or not when you explain it to them. There is nothing secretive about making mistakes and even fighting them–we all can give

34

examples—even his brothers and sisters. Explained in this way, it makes it easier for them to understand what they can do to be helpful. After all, if they were having difficulty learning an activity, they would want others (1) to give them time to work through their mistakes, (2) to wait calmly and not interrupt them or to jump in and do it for them. The same is true for a child who is stuttering (reacting to disruptions in his speech).

As a way to help, set up talking rules in your home. The talking rules apply to your child who stutters as well as to his brothers and sisters.

1) We don't interrupt each other as we are talking.
2) We take turns talking.
3) We don't talk for each other. Each does his own talking.

How should teasing be handled?

In addition to talking rules, I suggest that you establish a position about teasing. If discussions have been open about your child's stuttering problem, there should be a minimum of teasing. However, if teasing occurs by a brother or sister, it is easy to point out to them that if they worked hard on a math paper, for example, and then made many mistakes, they would feel badly. Anyone teasing them at that time would be very unkind. The same is true when they tease anyone else. You can set up a rule that in your family, one doesn't tease another about the way he or she does things. To do so, only makes one feel sad. It doesn't help one learn—and, we are a family and we are all trying to help each other.

What do I say to his friends?

Essentially, you can talk to them the same way I suggested you talk to his brothers and sisters. It is not unusual for a friend of your child to turn to you and ask "How come he talks that way?" or, "Why does he stutter?" Again, it is important that you answer in an open, matter-of-fact way. Your child will likely be present. Therefore you can give the same kind of explanation that you gave to your child and to his brothers and sisters. Presenting similar explanations about stuttering to your child's friends enables you to handle any teasing by friends in the same way explained previously for brothers and sisters.

What do I say to the baby sitter and to the people at the day care center?

I suggest that you explain to adults who take care of your child that he is stuttering some during this phase of learning to talk. You can reassure them that you want him to talk to them and you want them to talk to him. If you can help them view the stuttering as the making of mistakes, then it will be easier for them to see that he should be encouraged to express ideas just as any other child. You also can help them understand that when speech disruptions occur, the child should be given the time to work through them without listeners hurrying him or without their finishing words or ideas for him. At the same time, he should receive the same discipline practices as any other child. Also, he can be helped to learn the same talking manners as any other child. He should learn to "take turns" in talking and he should not interrupt, talk for, or finish words for anyone else – any more than they for him.

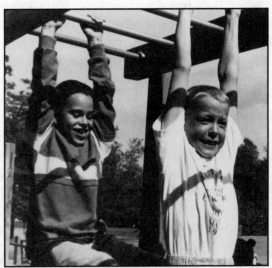

photo credit: paul diamond

What day care centers can do to help.

1) Treat the child who stutters the same as the other children at the center.
2) Don't let the child who stutters get away with things just because she stutters.
3) View the stuttering as making some mistakes in the normal learning process. This child should be encouraged to express ideas just as any other child at the center.
4) When she has disruptions in speech, allow her time to work through the mistakes.
   a) without listeners hurrying her
   b) without listeners finishing words or ideas for her.
5) The child who stutters should receive the same discipline as any other child.
6) The child who stutters should learn the same talking manners as any other child; for example, a) taking turns talking, b) listening while others talk, and c) not interrupting others or finishing their words or ideas for them.

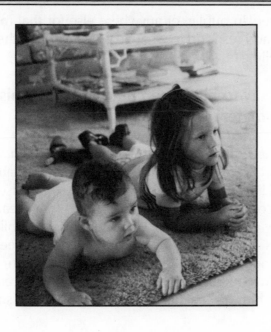

When his grandparents or his aunts and uncles ask, what should I say about his stuttering?

I suggest that you adopt the same basic philosophy with close relatives as I explained above under ways to talk to your own child and to his brothers and sisters about stuttering. This enables all close family members to see the problem in the same way. It provides a common-sense approach that is readily understandable and one that encourages all "family" to be consistent in the ways they react to the act of stuttering and to the child who is doing it.

What should I do if my child stutters in public and if a stranger comments about it?

I know that at times it may be difficult, but remember when a child stutters, he is talking–and when he is talking, he is trying–although clumsily at times–to send you a message. Therefore, attend to, and work to interpret the message. Don't get sidetracked by the static that may be accompanying the child's message.

If he stutters in public, or anywhere else for that matter, pay attention to and respond to what he is telling you rather than to how he is telling it.

What do I say to him when he is teased by his friends or his classmates?

Teasing is a common problem that most children have to deal with as a part of growing up. If they are not teased about their speech they likely will be teased about something else – for example, the color of their hair or the glasses they wear or even the way they eat a hamburger. Undoubtedly, your child will experience his share of teasing. In any event, he needs to be helped to understand about teasing generally. Then, it will be easier for him to figure out how to handle it. You can help by sharing with him his feelings about being teased. Also you can discuss together the things one can do when teased. You can even talk about the ways you felt and the things you did when you were teased as a child. Another thing you can do is to help him focus his attention on other things. For example, go for an ice cream cone, suggest he call a close friend, discuss plans for an upcoming event, and so forth.

As I talk to children about the teasing they do, they explain to me that they are not trying to be mean or to hurt one's feelings. They are just "kidding around." They say that they only "kid around" with their friends. They don't kid around with those they don't like or don't know. In my experience, most "teasing" is of this kind. You can work with your child to help him to decide the best way to handle it. If there is one child or a small group who tease to be cruel, then often it is best to discuss with the teacher, and, if necessary, the school counselor the best ways to handle it.

What do I say to his teachers?

I suggest that you make an appointment to meet your child's classroom teacher before classes begin. Teachers welcome the chance to discuss stuttering openly with parents. It will help the teacher to decide the most reasonable ways to handle your child's speech in the classroom if she learns how you have been handling it at home. She can appreciate the fact that you have talked to your child about bobbles and other disruptions in speech as "mistakes we make while learning to talk." Also, that the related physical tensing and struggling (if present) are efforts to fight or hide the mistakes. After all, the teacher's job is to help children learn. And she knows how upset some become when they don't do things "right."

The teacher will want to know that at home you encourage your child to say what he wants to say even though he has some disruptions while saying it. You react to what he says, not how he says it. You compliment him, not for speaking fluently, but for an interesting observation good talking manners in the home. No one interrupts, talks for or finishes words for anyone else.

You will want to learn from the teacher the kinds of oral recitation (oral reading, short answers, oral reports) the children perform. It will be helpful if you then talk about this with your child so he knows what to expect. Suggest to the teacher that she do the same thing. You both can learn the way he feels about it–the parts that don't worry him and the parts that do. Then you and the teacher can discuss the best ways to help him meet constructively oral recitations. There are certain activities that have been found to be helpful to other children. These include–

(a) If the child is fearful of reciting orally, his reading assignments can be sent home. You can have him practice reading them alone to you. This enables him to gain confidence of knowing all of the words, and it gives him the experience of hearing his voice as he reads.

(b) If he is afraid of being asked questions to be answered aloud, you can pretend to be the teacher and ask him to answer questions aloud. This enables him to practice taking the time to answer, to revise an answer, and generally to "think on his feet" out loud.

(c) If he is afraid of activities involving telling a story or giving an oral report, he can prepare it and present it to you–and perhaps to other members of the family.

If the teacher knows the things you are doing, she can plan her activities with the child accordingly. The important goal to be reached is for the teacher to ask him to recite just as she does any other child in the classroom.

If speech therapy is recommended, indicate to the speech clinician and to the teacher that you will cooperate in every way possible.

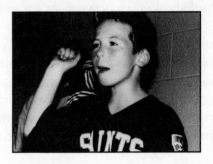

Things that you as a teacher can do to help.

1) Meeting with parents of a child who stutters before or near the beginning of classes will help you learn the parents' concerns and expectations.
2) If there is a speech clinician at your school, contact her to see what suggestions she may have for this child. If she is working with him, find out what her objectives are.
3) Encourage good talking manners in the classroom: no one interrupts, talks for or finishes words for anyone else.
4) Don't let the child who stutters get away with things just because he stutters.
5) As much as possible, treat the child who stutters the same as the other children in your class - with the exception of special assistance with oral recitation.
6) Children who stutter should be expected to perform all classroom oral recitations even though they may need some special help to succeed.
7) Talk with the child about the class's oral recitation requirements, how he feels about it and what you can do to help.
8) Give and encourage the child a chance to practice his oral recitation requirements at home.
9) Allow children who stutter enough time to talk; they may frequently have trouble starting to talk.
10) Know that your caring enough to do these things can make a big difference!

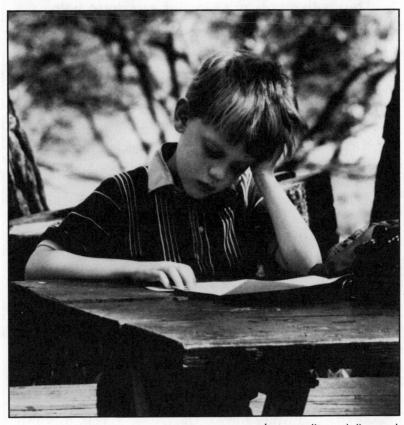

photo credit: paul diamond

Chapter 5

what is involved in therapy?

Hugo H. Gregory, Ph.D.
Professor, Director of Stuttering Programs
Speech and Language Pathology Program
Northwestern University

Therapy may consist of a few sessions with parents or it may involve a longer relationship of working with both the parents and the child for several months. In general, the older the child, the longer therapy will take. With a preschool child, the clinician tries to prevent or minimize stuttering. The older the child when therapy begins, the less likely all traces of the problem can be eliminated. This chapter provides information about what is involved in therapy and deals with questions you may have about how therapy can help.

How are decisions made about what is needed?

In general, deciding what a child needs in therapy involves: (1) the ways in which your child's speech differs from that of most children, and (2) what circumstances in his speech development or environment are contributing to the problem.

Specifically, we are more concerned about a child who has more (1) one syllable word repetitions ("I,I,I" "He,He,He") and/or (2) breaks within words (sound repetitions "M,M,M,Mama," syllable repetitions "Mamamamama," sound prolongations "MMMMama") Noticeable tension (that may be seen or heard) in the lips, jaw, larynx or chest areas accompanying these repetitions and prolongations, or blocks in the child's speech, are more certain signs of a stuttering problem.

If stuttering has been present for more than six months, and if it is becoming more constant from day to day, and more consistent from one situation to the next, more than just parent guidance is likely to be recommended.

If stress in the way the parents and others talk to the child or stress in the way family members relate to each other is contributing to increased stuttering, then these stresses must be reduced.

Circumstances That May Increase Stuttering

Communicative Stress	Interpersonal Stress
The Way Parents and Others Talk with the Child	The Way Family Members Relate to Each Other
1. Rapid speech rates and fast paced conversation	1. Unrealistic demands on the child
2. Interrupting the child	2. Conflict about discipline
3. Guessing what the child is about to say	3. Hectic or inconsistent family routine
4. Beginning to speak immediately when the child pauses or stops talking.	4. Fast paced family life
5. Bombarding the child with many questions	5. Experiences that make the child feel "put down"
6. Competing to get into a conversation	

Some children who stutter may also have other speech problems; they may have trouble pronouncing some sounds or words or they may have trouble choosing words quickly and correctly. Since these other speech problems could be related to the development of stuttering or could complicate treatment, therapy focuses on these problems as well when it is appropriate.

At what age should a child be evaluated or receive therapy?

Ordinarily, parents don't get concerned about a child's speech–"Is my child beginning to stutter?"–until at least 24 to 36 months of age, when the child uses sufficient language to speak in sentences. Whenever parents are concerned about a child's speech, it is time to see a speech clinician who works with children. If it is a question about stuttering, parents should seek one who includes stuttering as one of the areas in which he/she is specialized.

How can I tell if my child knows he is stuttering?

A child just beginning to stutter may say "Why can't I talk?" or "I can't say it." We cannot be sure just what this means in terms of awareness. But if he talks about it several times a week, he is probably becoming more aware. If the child stops talking when he is having trouble or changes his speech in some way, for example by whispering, this is a more certain sign that he knows he is stuttering.

There is nothing wrong with occasionally commenting about obvious speech difficulty by saying, "All people have trouble talking sometimes. You are still learning how to talk." Or you may say, "Talking seems a little harder for you today." It is important to acknowledge the difficulty the child is experiencing.

How are parents involved in therapy?

Since the home environment has a very strong influence on the child's speech, it is clear that the parents are going to be involved in therapy.

Early in the process, we find that parents have many questions about speech development and stuttering. We describe the development of speech from words to phrases to sentences, and help them to identify the ways in which the smooth flow of speech may be disrupted (sound repetitions or prolongations, syllable repetitions, blocks, etc.)

As the parents describe those situations that seem to increase or decrease their child's stuttering, we instruct them how to chart episodes of increased stuttering. The following chart illustrates this procedure.

Situation	What Did the Child Do?	Child's Speech	Child's Awareness	Cause of Child's Speech Disruption	What Did Parents Do?
Mother & Father are talking	Interrupted. Wanted Father's attention	Repeated syllables prolonged sounds in tense way	Excited, but unaware of speech problems	The child wants immediate attention can't wait.	Father said "I'll listen as soon as your mother & I are through talking." And he did.

In the illustration above we worked with parents for better ways to manage the situation. Here, the speech clinician suggested having "talking times" with the child. Then the parents were advised to have times at home in which Mother and Father listened carefully to the child and emphasized each having a turn to talk. When the child did this too, he was encouraged by being told, "I like the way you are taking turns." As progress was made, taking turns was discussed with other family members. The goal was to give the child more attention in a structured way and to help him learn how to take part in a conversation without interrupting others.

46

We as speech clinicians not only tell but also show the parents what changes to make. We may demonstrate a more relaxed, slightly slower rate of speaking, pausing longer after the child speaks before responding. Gradually, parents take over more of the clinician's role and use the changed behavior when talking with the child. Children respond better when they know that their parents are learning too.

Isn't it hard for parents to change their behavior?

Yes it is, and it is also very important. This is why the clinician arranges for changes to be made in small steps and provides opportunities for practice at the clinic before any attempt is made to make changes at home. In a group session, parents often share with other parents some of their questions, frustrations, and successes. Most parents want to learn to respond appropriately, and once they get into the process of change, it is rewarding. The best reward for the parents is to see their child's speech improving.

How does the clinician work with the child?

Pre-school age children

When a child is seen in the very early stages of beginning to stutter, parent guidance (or counseling) only will usually be the approach used. Some clinicians want to always take a look at changing the child's environment before working more directly with the child. Some suggest permissive, warm, sharing, comfortable speaking situations in the clinic along with parent guidance. Additional observations of the child can be made in this atmosphere which is usually conducive to more relaxed speech.

The clinician makes a decision about more direct therapy with the child taking into into consideration:

1) the amount of tension in the child's speech,
2) how long the problem has existed,
3) how constant the condition is, and

4) whether or not there are other related problems of speech.

For example, if the problem has been present for less than a year, stuttering is still what we call a borderline problem, and there are no complicating speech problems, then the child may be seen on a short term basis (4 to 10 sessions). The parents can watch the clinician working with the child and can do such things as those listed below:

1. Talk in a calmer, slower and more relaxed way.

2. Pause about 2 or 3 seconds after the child finishes speaking before responding.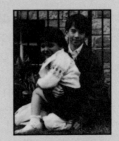

3. Make a point of commenting on what the child says, not the way he says it.

4. Ask fewer questions. When questions are asked, ask one at a time and give the child ample time to answer.

5. Most of all, encourage each person in the family to listen to the other. When one speaks, the other listens, then takes his/her turn.

Recently, when a father saw me doing this with his child, he said, "I know I have always been energetic and excited when playing with Tony. I thought that was the way to get his interest. I just never thought about how that could be related to his stuttering."

When the pattern of stuttering is more firmly established, even in preschool children, the clinician may help these children change their speech by showing them (modeling) an easier, more relaxed manner of speaking beginning with shorter and working up to longer utterances. To get the most out of therapy, parents must learn to model for the child, just like the clinician does.

School Age Children

With older school children, the clinician can be more direct in showing the child how to reduce tension and speak in a more easy relaxed way with smooth movements between words. Of course, therapy is different with each child. Often, just showing the child–beginning with words and working up to longer phrases–how to speak in a slower, more relaxed manner is enough. With others, we may contrast "easy talking" with "hard talking", and in those where there is more tension (and expectation of difficulty) on certain sounds or words, we help the child to be more aware of tension and contrast this with the easier more relaxed way. As one eight-year-old youngster said to me, "I can tell my speech what to do."

The school age child's attitudes are dealt with in two ways: (1) by explaining to them how speech is produced and by helping them to see that changing speech is like learning a skill in a sport (hitting a ball) and, (2) by being a good listener and helping the child deal with his worries and concerns, such as teasing by a peer.

Are there drugs that will help?

No! Since tension is obviously involved in stuttering, there has been substantial interest in the use of tranquilizers and relaxants in the treatment of stuttering. Research will continue, but at present there is agreement among speech clinicians and medical specialists that drug therapy is not effective.

Are there devices that stop a person's stuttering?

The speech of some stutterers improves when they speak while listening to a rather intense noise through earphones. This change may be due to stutterers not being able to hear their own voice, thus reducing learned cues associated with the habit of stuttering. Research shows that the noise causes the person to speak more loudly and prolong sounds somewhat, and it is believed that this may also contribute to increased fluency.

The advent of the Edinburgh Masker has increased the interest of clinicians and stutterers in this masking effect. This instrument consists of a voice-activated microphone that is worn snugly fitted to the larynx so that when the person speaks, a "humming" noise is delivered through hearing aid type earphones worn in the ears. The Edinburgh Masker has been especially beneficial to those adults who have attempted speech modification procedures with little success. Since it must be worn to be effective,it is recommended that adult stutterers have therapy aimed toward modifying their speech before resorting to the masker. The use of this device is not the therapy of choice with children. They have not been found willing to wear it. Also, since there is hope of preventing a problem, or minimizing the difficulty using the procedures described above, use of the masker with children is not advisable. However, some clinicians may use a masking noise as an adjunct to more conventional therapy with a school age child.

A delayed auditory feedback device may be used in therapy to help a school age child experience increased fluency or to counter certain bad habits of speaking. The child's speech is recorded immediately and played back through earphones with a very brief delay (about 1/5 of a second). Ordinarily, this delay disrupts a child's speech, but if the clinician instructs the child who stutters to prolong speech sounds slightly and to speak a little slower, the child stutters less, but the child's speech often sounds monotonous and un-natural.

What about the parents' role in therapy at school?

School speech clinicians often say that it is difficult to do successful therapy in the schools because they cannot counsel parents as needed. Children are so much more successful when they have their parents' support and realize that their Mother and Father know what they are doing in therapy. Parents can learn to reinforce what their child is learning. The school speech clinician, the teachers, and the parents should be a team in working with the school age child who stutters.

How much therapy is needed?

This depends on the many factors described above. When a decision has been made to see both parents and child for therapy, it is best for therapy to be fairly intensive at first, that is at least three individual sessions of 30-50 minutes a week. The frequency of therapy is reduced as the child improves.

How long will it take?

It may only take a few weeks with a preschool child just beginning to stutter. With a more developed problem in either a preschool or school age child, therapy may take up to eighteen months, sometimes more. Since so many circumstances affect speech, it is important that children be followed carefully for several years following therapy. During this time, the parents and the clinician should stay in touch. In this way, therapy for a child who stutters could last a long time.

When is consultation with another professional, such as a psychologist, needed?

In discussing the environment of the child, we have referred to interpersonal stress related to increased stuttering. Some examples of these stress factors are:

1) Parents who have unrealistic levels of expectation for their children's behavior such as neatness and table manners (oftentimes these parents have high levels of expectation for speech development).

2) Sibling rivalries or discipline practices that are causing conflict.

3) Hectic or inconsistent family routines.

4) Parents who are anxious about child rearing practices or have feelings of guilt about how they have reacted to their child's speech.

5) Some basic unhappiness in a marriage.

When the speech clinician sees that stress factors such as these are consistently interfering with progress in therapy, a referral to a psychologist (preferably one interested in children with speech problems) for evaluation may provide helpful insight or indicate that another treatment such as family therapy or psychotherapy for the child or parents is needed. Often times, such a referral leads to a more positive outcome. Sometimes parents do not accept this advice. Some clinics employ a multidisciplinary approach in which the child who stutters and parents are always seen by a psychologist. Circumstances surrounding a stuttering problem in a child are often fairly complex, and input from other professionals is often helpful.

How much success can be expected?

Success rates are very high when therapy begins during the period of two and one half to five years of age. They are even better when parents have taken proper steps when they were first concerned. With school age children, it is less likely that fluency can be completely normalized. If the child reacts with frustration to the therapy process, it may be best to postpone treatment until later. If the child does not appear to be benefiting from therapy, the speech clinician should be able to explain why, and you should have the kind of relationship with the clinician in which the reasons can be discussed freely. Consultation with another clinician should be considered.

Who should we go to for therapy?

You should seek a speech clinician who includes stuttering as one of the areas in which he/she is specialized. More and more clinicians are specializing in stuttering. Talk to more than one professional before you choose. When you have narrowed your choices, consult with some of the clinicians' colleagues about their reputations. This is an important decision. It involves your time and your money, and most of all your child's future.

How much will therapy cost?

Private practitioners charge from forty to ninety dollars per hour. Most often the fee will be sixty-five to seventy-five dollars an hour. Total cost could be from one to several thousand dollars. Of course, in the case of short term treatment such as that described for some children beginning to stutter, it could be less. You should be satisfied with progress as therapy proceeds and feel free to inquire about the prognosis and costs. Therapy in university clinics, where students are being trained, or in publicly supported institutions, is less expensive. Health insurance policy coverage of stuttering therapy varies. You should consult with your agent and request that the speech clinician send reports or any other required information to the company.

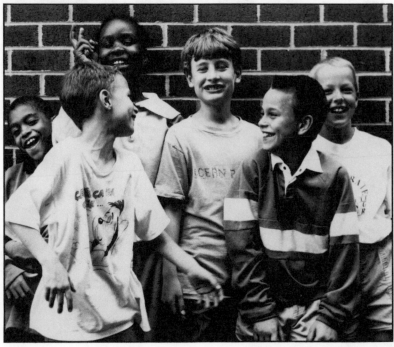

photo credit: paul diamond

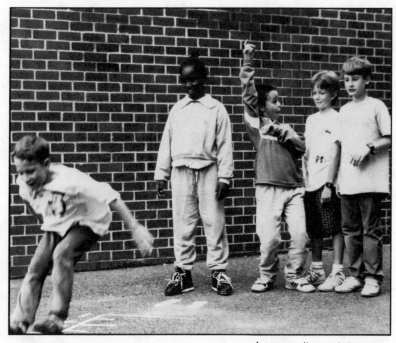

photo credit: paul diamond

Chapter 6

what if my child continues to stutter?

Barry Guitar, Ph.D.
Professor, Department of Communication
Science and Disorders
University of Vermont

If your child's stuttering persists after treatment, you may have questions about how it will affect him. You may wonder how it will influence his social development and his school achievement as well as his future happiness. You may also want to know what you can do that will help. Our answers to these questions, given in this section, are based on experiences with many children with a wide variety of stuttering problems. The vast majority of these children have continued to improve their speech as they grew older, with the help and support of their parents.

What should I do if he still stutters after therapy?

Therapy with young children can result in stuttering's being cured or reduced so much that it is hardly noticeable. If your child has had therapy and has improved, he may still slip from time to time, however. For example, your child may stutter a little when he is excited or tired. Be accepting of some slippage. Even if he slips a lot, show him you really care about him apart from whether he stutters or not, by listening attentively to his message and ignoring the stuttering.

If your child is stuttering mildly, and for brief periods, it isn't likely to bother him. He will probably be able to handle it, especially if you are supportive. On the other hand, if your child is stuttering enough so that he is tensing pretty hard to get words out, or is avoiding talking, he may need further therapy. If you aren't sure, check with the therapist who worked with him before.

Sometimes, going back for a booster session will be enough to get him back on track. Other times, going to a different therapist may be appropriate. See how your child feels about it.

Will continued stuttering hinder his academic success?

Many brilliant scientists and writers–for example, Charles Darwin and Lewis Carroll–were stutterers. Thus there is no reason to suppose that stuttering is caused by low intelligence or is associated with poor achievement. In fact, a great many stutterers take pride in how well they did in school and college. Your child's success in school will be influenced by many individual factors, independent of stuttering, such as how bright he is or how motivated he is. His academic success will probably be greater if he doesn't let his stuttering keep him from participating in class. Good teachers can make a difference in this regard, too. They can encourage your child to talk despite his stuttering, and they can help him realize that others appreciate his ideas. It is important, therefore, that you and the school clinician stay in contact with your child's teachers to help them foster his school progress. Through this contact, you and the clinician can also inform teachers who may not understand stuttering or know how to react appropriately to it.

If your child chooses to go to college, his stuttering will not keep him from doing so. College admissions officers are likely to welcome a student who has experienced a problem like stuttering, but hasn't let it hold him back. Many colleges and universities, in fact, provide speech therapy services because they expect that some of their students will stutter or have other speech disorders.

Will stuttering keep him from making friends?

No. Making friends is done by being friendly. Your child may find it a little harder to talk to other kids his age, but as long as he does talk in a friendly way with others, he will have friends.

Many of the children who stutter that I know have plenty of friends because they are a lot of fun. They like other people and they have a good sense of humor. They don't let their stuttering keep them from being talkative and playful.

I have worked with kids who stuttered only a little, but were at first so worried about their stuttering that they didn't talk a lot. Their parents worried too, and that didn't help. As we worked together, these kids loosened up. They learned to be less bothered when they were teased about their stuttering. They talked about their stuttering to other kids. They also began to get interested in other kids, which naturally led to making friends.

Will my child be able to play sports?

Absolutely. Some of the most talented athletes of this decade are stutterers. For example, Bob Love, Lester Hayes, and Bill Walton are all stutterers as well as superstars. Of course very few of us are going to be that talented. But if your child likes to play sports, he'll find it rewarding. If he's good, or just enthusiastic, other kids will enjoy playing sports with him. That, in turn, will boost his confidence, which may help his speech.

Children who stutter often feel most free when they are able to lose themselves in something that doesn't focus on speech, like sports or other physical activities. Stuttering often disappears or becomes very mild when a child plays sports. Even a severe stutterer can usually yell just about anything to his team mates during the excitement of a game.

What does the future hold if his stuttering persists into adolescence and beyond?

You may be thinking far into the future, wondering about whether your child would have any problems dating, marrying, or bringing up children. The answer is that he will probably have no more problems than someone who doesn't stutter.

Let's begin with the first step in the sequence. Dating, for teenagers, can be hard at first, whether they stutter or not. Most teenagers who stutter learn to go ahead and make friends with members of the opposite sex despite their stuttering. They find out that if they are friendly, their approach is usually successful. Whether a real relationship develops is a matter of chemistry and common interests. Stuttering doesn't get in the way once two people get to know each other. Nor does it get in the way of a relationship that leads to marriage.

Stuttering is also no barrier to having a happy marriage and raising a family. It is true that children of stutterers may inherit an increased vulnerability to stuttering, but most will not stutter. Even if they do, parents who stutter themselves usually know what responses are most helpful to a child who may begin to stutter. They have good ideas about how to talk about stuttering with their children. They can be objective and can share feelings about stuttering. They can create a home environment that nurtures the growth of fluent speech.

You may wonder if your child's stuttering will become more of a problem as he grows older in other ways than marriage and a family. Perhaps you know someone who stutters severely and for whom stuttering is a problem relating to people or talking to the public. It is important for you to know that it doesn't have to be this way. For example, I stutter on many occasions, but I speak in public, meet new people easily, talk on the telephone, do all the things that completely fluent speakers do. Most of the time I speak fairly easily, but occasionally I get hung up on a stutter. My listeners usually take their cues from how I react. When I keep my cool despite stuttering, my listeners hardly notice the stuttering. Sure, some people are impatient, but I have learned not to let them get me down.

There are days when stuttering does get in my way. I go through periods when my stuttering flares up for reasons I don't always understand. I sometimes avoid words I might stutter on or situations that are hard for me when I know I shouldn't. Sometimes I might feel discouraged. This aspect of stuttering is a real annoyance, but it is something I have learned to deal with. Most other adult stutterers learn to deal with it too.

What can I do that will help my child now?

If your child's stuttering persists after therapy, there are things you can do that will help him. Perhaps the most important advice we can give you is what we have said before: be accepting of your child if his stuttering returns. Try to find out if there are new stresses or a return of old ones. Try to recall if there were things that you were doing when your child was in therapy. Perhaps you have forgotten some of the things that were helpful–for example, speaking slowly and easily when talking to your child. Can you do those again? For more specific ideas, read the book, *If Your Child Stutters: A Guide for Parents.* If you have read it before, reread the latest edition for reminders of what you can do to help your child.

Although you are probably one of the most important influences on how your child responds to his stuttering, there may be other people who affect your child's stuttering and his feelings. One example is people who are impatient with him because of his stuttering. Sometimes you can speak to them in private to change their behavior. Many times, however, you can't intervene in time. But you always have the opportunity to let your child know he's OK as he is, whether he stutters or not.

If he is having a particularly bad time with his stuttering, he may feel down in the dumps. You can help a lot here by encouraging him to talk about how he feels. Your child may feel frustrated or angry or hurt because of his stuttering. Being able to share these feelings can make it easier for him. Try to sense what he's feeling by his facial expression and tone of voice. Share with him that you also have had temporary feelings of sadness or anger.

When your child's stuttering bothers you, and it surely will on some days, try to remember that some of his reactions to it are determined by those around him. If you can foster an acceptance of the stuttering in your family, your child will be likely to struggle with it less and less. He will learn to talk confidently in spite of it.

In Summary

If your child still stutters after therapy, you can help him in several ways. First, be accepting of your child even if his stuttering bothers you. Show your caring, especially when his stuttering seems worst. That is when he needs you most. Second, encourage your child in all ways to be himself. Your efforts will show him that stuttering is only one part of his life.

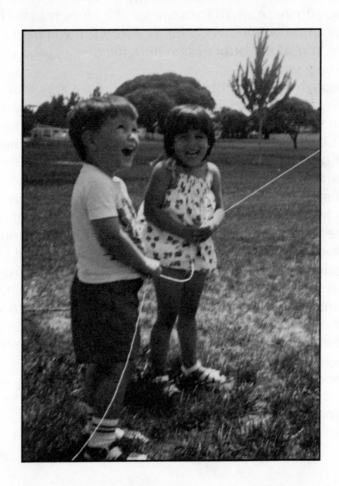

Chapter 7

should we seek help?

William H. Perkins, Ph.D.
Professor Emeritus, Communication Arts and Sciences,
Otolaryngology, and Speech Science and Technology
University of Southern California

Won't therapy make him more aware of his problem? Make his problem worse?

For years, everyone (many professionals included) tiptoed around stuttering as if we were walking on eggs for fear of calling attention to the problem. Many presumed that this would make it worse. No longer. You should consider two things.

For one thing, if your child's stuttering is developing into a problem for him, he is already becoming aware of it and is frustrated by it. When parents pretend nothing is wrong, he may conclude that his stuttering is so bad they can't even talk about it.

The second consideration is that early treatment has shown the best results of all. Instead of making stuttering worse, the sooner effective help is provided after stuttering is first noticed, the better the child's chances of full recovery. If stuttering continues after puberty, it usually persists in one form or another.

Will he be cured?

If stuttering does persist into adulthood, he may dream of cure, but hardly anyone, neither professionals nor people who stutter, realistically expects anything more than improvements. These adults may be able to sound normal much of the time, but most continue to think of themselves as stutterers.

With children, the prospects are much better. By helping them before they begin to fear stuttering and develop reactions to it–

fear and reactions which complicate the lives of adults who stutter-these children have a good chance of becoming at least reasonably normal speakers. They may still stumble and hesitate in their speech from time to time, but that happens to everyone. The important thing is that these children not feel so frustrated by their bobbles that speaking becomes a struggle and they begin to identify themselves as stutterers. Prevention of a self-image of being a stutterer goes a long way towards what could be called a cure for stuttering. Beginning therapy as soon as the problem becomes apparent goes a long way towards prevention.

Where do we begin to seek help?

First you need to find a specialist who has up-to-date knowledge of stuttering. Although any speech clinician licensed by the state or certified by the American Speech-Language-Hearing Association has at least minimal qualification to provide professional help for stuttering, most refer this problem to clinicians who have specialized in it. For much the same reason even though legally qualified, most licensed physicians who have not specialized in surgery refer patients to a surgeon. Likewise, most speech clinicians refer for specialized problems like stuttering. Universities and colleges with training programs in speech pathology (communication disorders) will be able to direct you to such specialists, as will the Speech Foundation of America, which is devoted exclusively to serving the interests of people who stutter.

What do I ask my pediatrician? Whose advice should we take?

Pediatricians have specialized knowledge of the health problems of children, so all questions concerning your child's health should be directed to them. Stuttering, however, is not a problem about which most physicians have adequate information, but they usually know a speech clinician to whom they routinely refer a wide variety of speech and language disorders. However, you would be well advised to determine if these speech clinicians are successful in treating children who stutter. If they are not, then ask them for a referral to someone who is.

What if I'm told that my child who stutters will "outgrow it?"

The chances are good that he will. Fifty to eighty percent of children whose parents think they have stuttered will stop before adulthood, and most of these before puberty.

It's the risk that your child may be one of the 20% to 50% that won't that you need to consider. First, was it a specialist in stuttering who told you he is "likely to outgrow it?" That prediction is difficult to make. It requires expert knowledge and experience.

The reason you may want to begin therapy early, rather than wait, is that his chances of full recovery dwindle the older he grows. If in doubt, you have much to gain and little to lose by starting treatment as early as possible.

If we are uncomfortable with the help, should we seek a second opinion?

Yes. You would be wise to seek a second opinion even if you're not uncomfortable with the first. And if you're still uncomfortable seek a third opinion. Diagnosis and treatment are far from being exact sciences. Even the best authorities have honest differences of opinion, so it pays to find out what more than one expert thinks.

If therapy is recommended, can he receive it at school?

Many schools do have clinicians who work successfully with children who stutter. Compared to the frequency of occurrence of other speech and language disorders, school clinicians see stuttering relatively infrequently, so they may not have much experience treating children who stutter.

Here are two suggestions for finding out if your school clinician can provide the necessary help. The first is to ask the parents of a stuttering child, who was treated by your potential clinician, what their experience was. The other is to try the therapy at school.

How soon will we know if he's being helped? What should we look for?

With young children, positive changes begin to appear sometimes within weeks, certainly within several months. What you need to look for are signs of gradual improvement, not a quick cure. As long as he is feeling better about himself, about his speech, and increasingly enjoys talking, you are on the right track. If he continues to struggle to speak, to avoid certain words and situations, to not want to talk at school or at home – these are signs that therapy is not helping much. Give it a fair trial, at least several months, before passing judgment.

Will he have to go every day?

Intensive therapy (three or more times a week) has advantages, so if the opportunity for frequent therapy is available, take it. This is especially true for older children at the beginning of treatment. Later sessions can be spaced farther apart without slowing progress.

Intensive therapy may not be available, however, especially at school. This certainly doesn't mean it won't be successful, but it does mean it will probably take longer.

———— • ————

No matter how long your child receives therapy, chances are very good it will help. Together with your love and guidance, there is every reason to believe that your child can be helped to become a more fluent speaker. For additional advice on how you can help, read *If Your Child Stutters: A Guide for Parents,* available from the Stuttering Foundation of America.